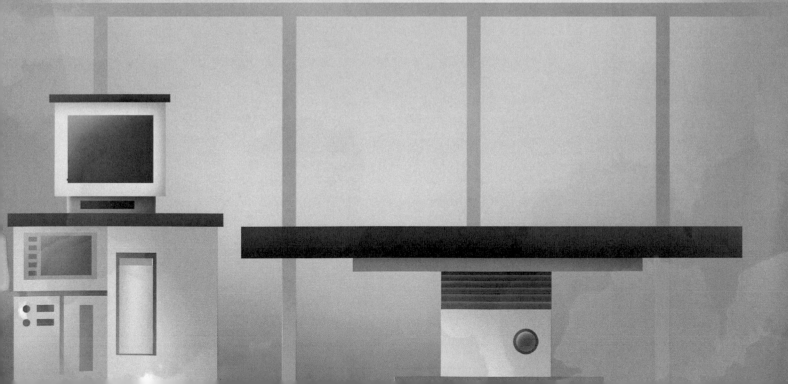

LITTLE MAN

Goes to

SURGERY!

Publisher: That's Love Publishing LLC
Printed in the United States of America.
ISBN 978-1953751-26-3

First printing, 2022.
Orders by U.S. trade bookstores and wholesalers
Please contact Erica Basora
at erica@thatslovepublishing.com
Website: thatslovepublishing.com

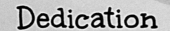

Dedication

This book is dedicated to all the children that find themselves having surgery. You are brave, courageous, and you can do this!
To my preceptor who gave me the tools and encouragement to keep going and helped me become the circulator I am today. I am so very grateful for your support and love.
To my Operating Room family, thank you for being a part of my team and impacting the lives of many daily. Many will never see what happens behind the red line, but they will be affected by your dedication and hard work. You all are amazing!

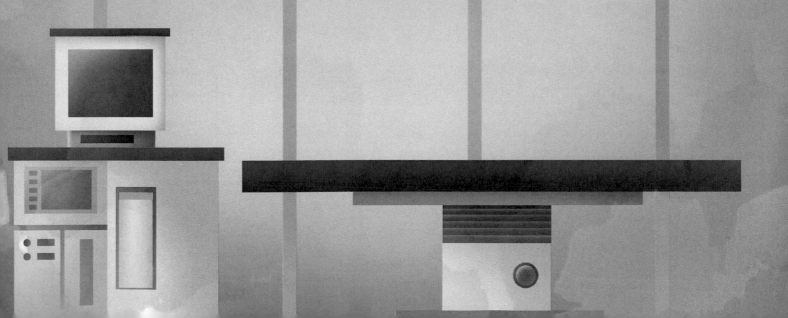

"Little Man, HELLO!"
"Hi Pop Pop! It is almost time for me to go!"
"Are you ready for your big day?"
"Well, I am a little nervous, I have to say."

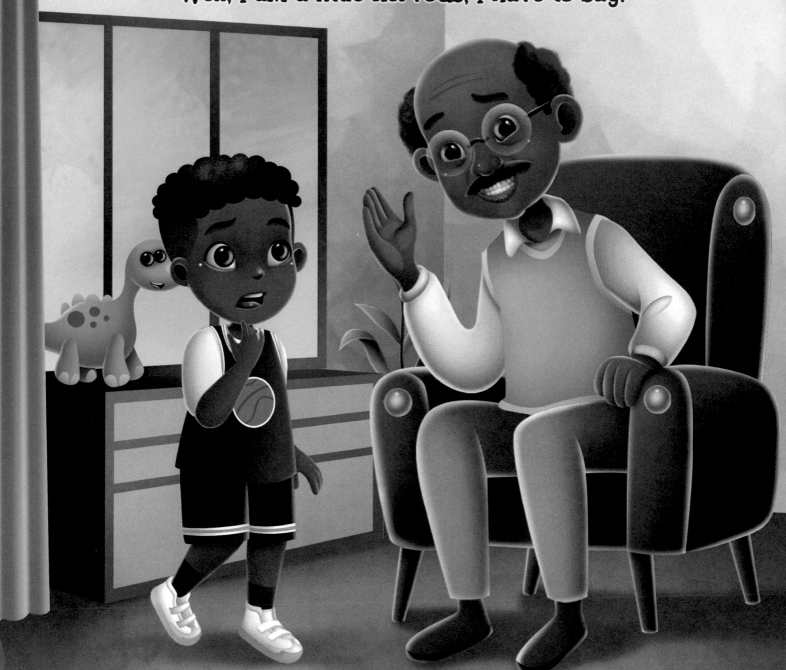

Mom makes sure we have all our things, like underwear,
And I cannot forget Danny, my favorite stuffed dinosaur.
He keeps me safe and sound and feeling sure,
He is my best friend and his love is pure.

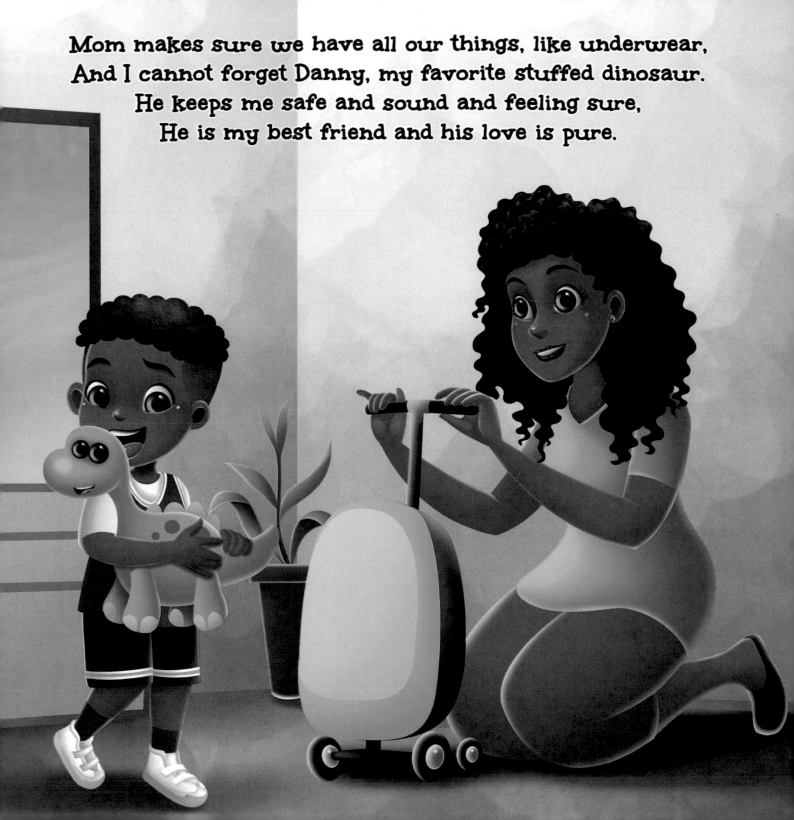

Time to give Baby Sis and Pop Pop a kiss,
It is them I will definitely miss.
I blow a kiss as I run to the car,
The drive to the hospital will not be too far.

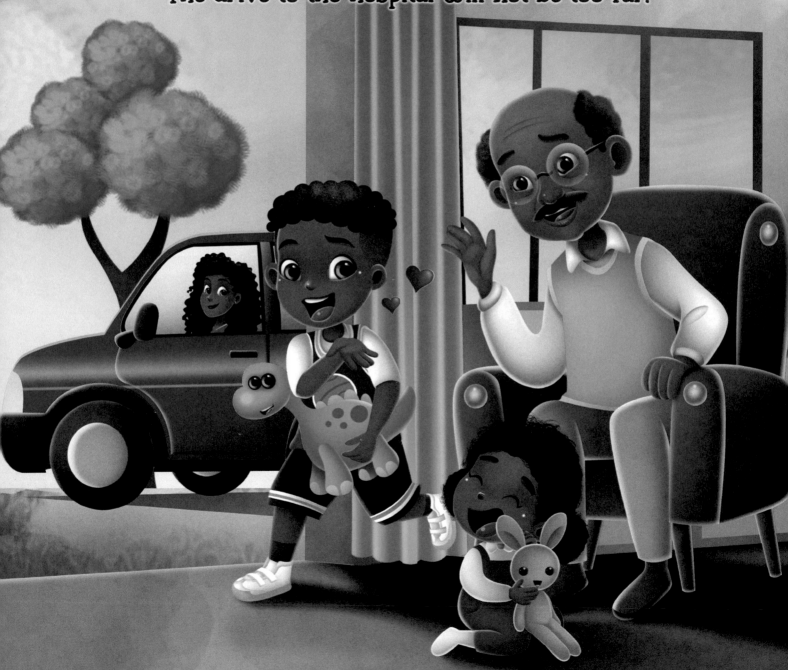

In the car Mom tries to chat.
Not in the mood, I feel shy as a cat.
"Little Man, are you okay?"
"Yes Mom, just not a lot to say."
"You know that everything will be okay?"
"Yes Mom, just keeping my thoughts on the day."

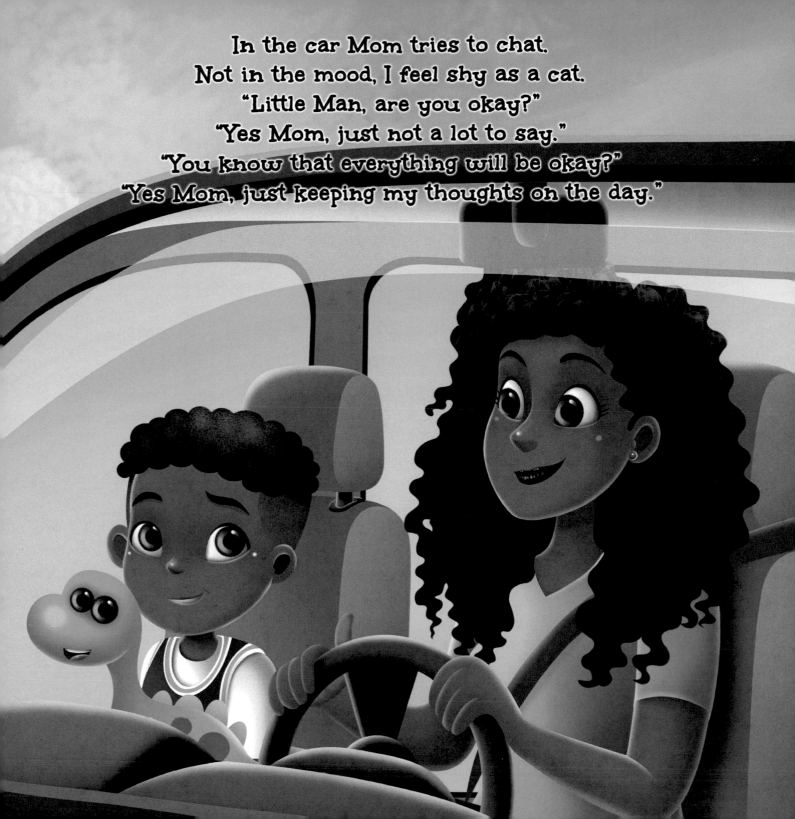

We get to the hospital and everything is so bright,
A friendly smile greets us and points us to the right.
A corner full of toys is where Danny and I go to play,
A Child Specialist comes over and says, "Little Man, may I join you today?"

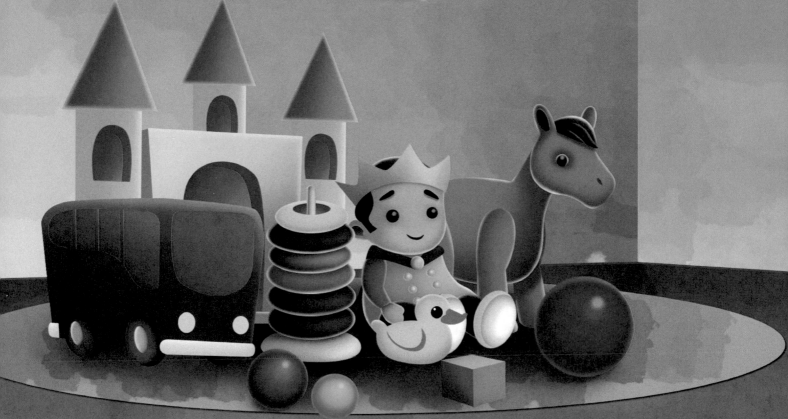

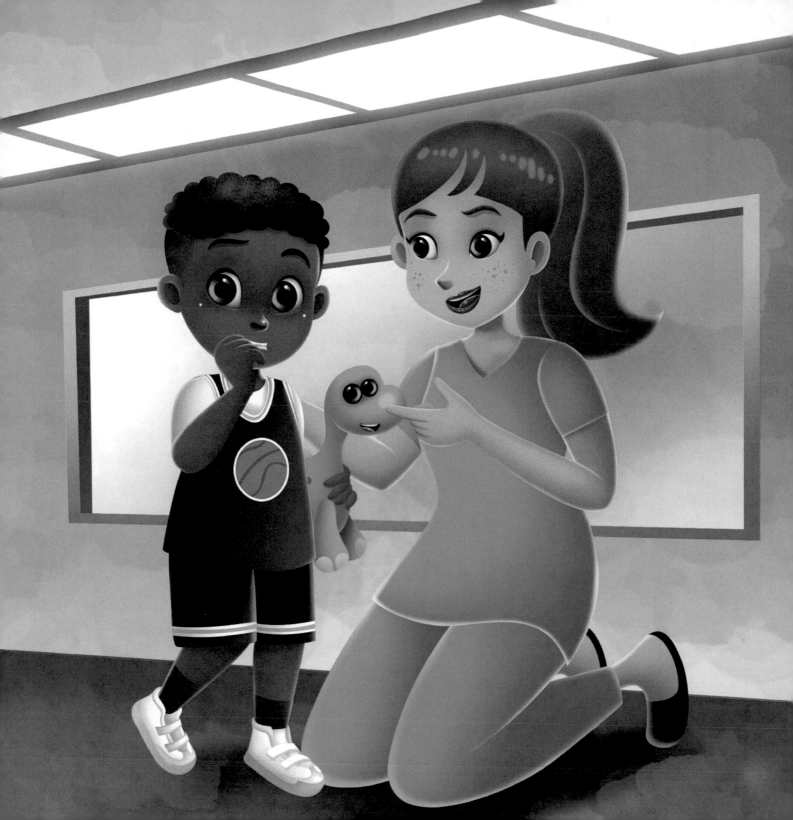

"Hi, my name is Mrs. Jen and I am here for you,
Do you have questions or worries or need to go to the loo?"
"I am nervous and scared and feeling blue,
But I know that surgery is the answer to being good as new."

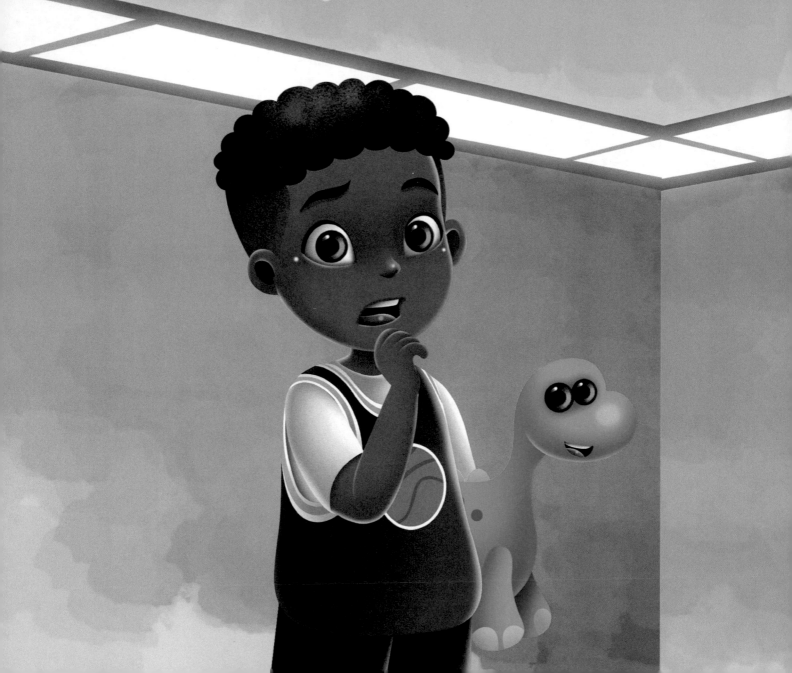

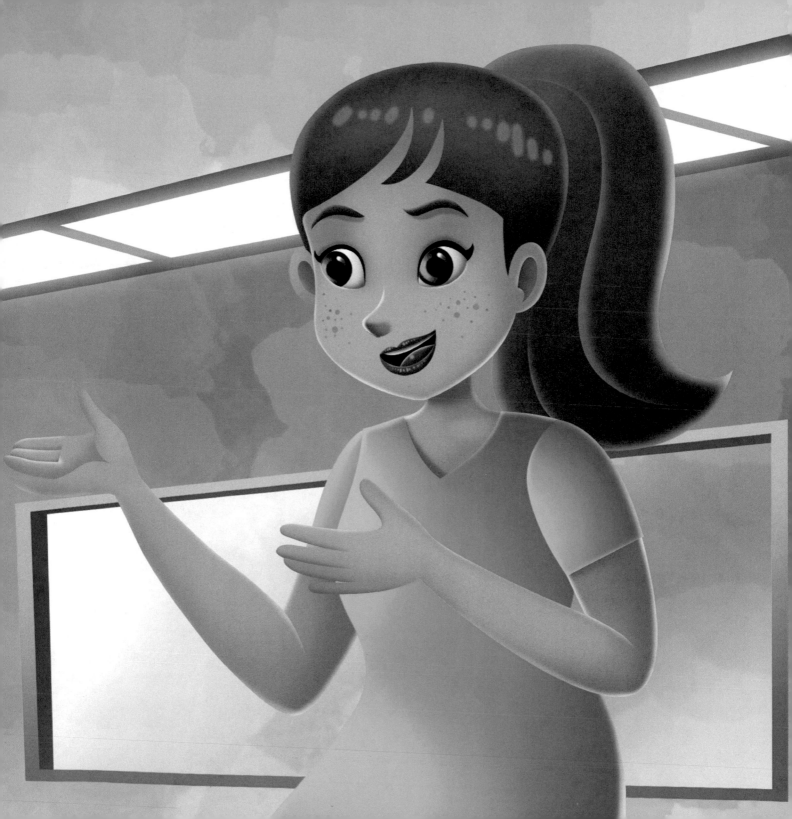

Mrs. Jen brings out a doll to show me what is happening next,
This doll looks just like me! That is THE BEST!
"Little Man, you will go to a room where Nurse Becky will be,
She will get you ready for surgery
with a gown and blanket, you'll see.
After that, you will get a fancy straw in your hand, which is an IV."

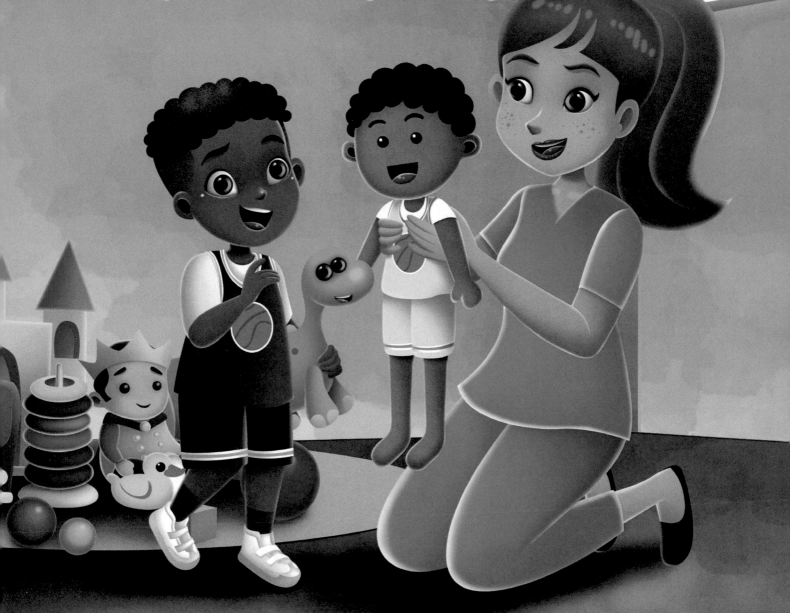

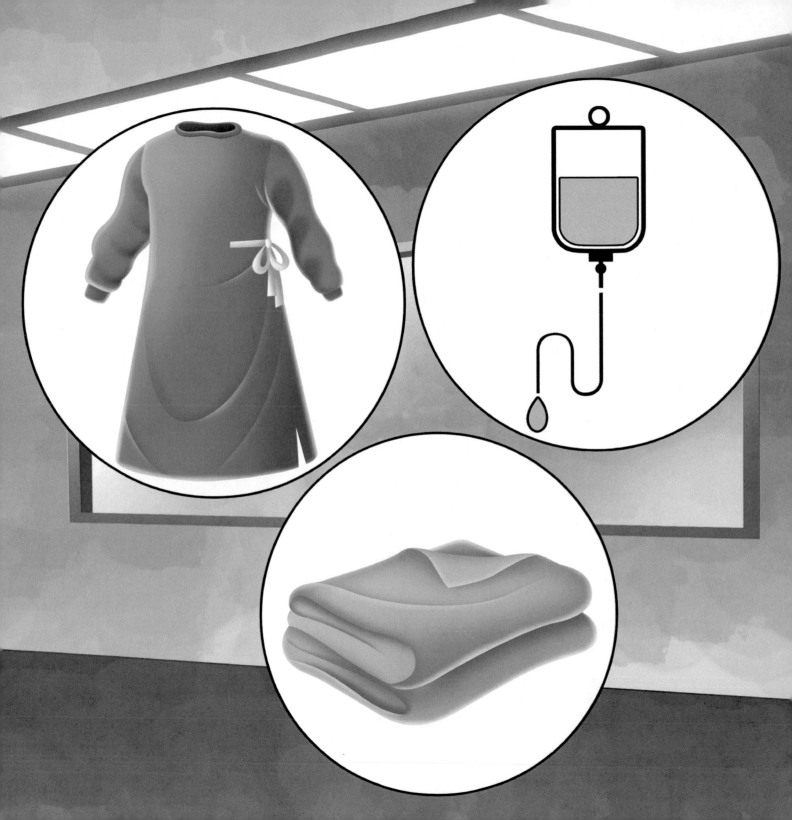

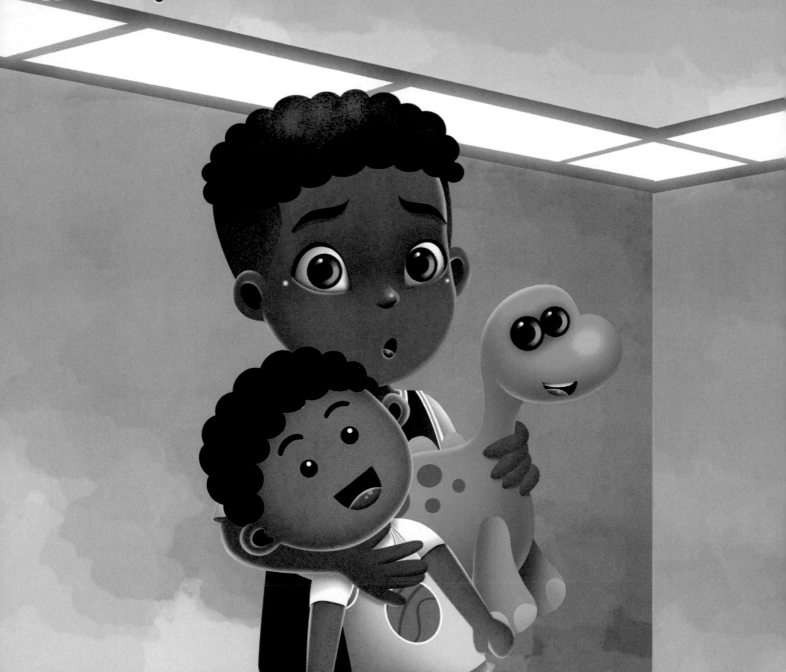

"Will it hurt?"
"It feels like a pinch, you have felt worse.
After that, you will get a hat to keep your head warm
And then you will chat with Dr. Serrano, she is there to inform."

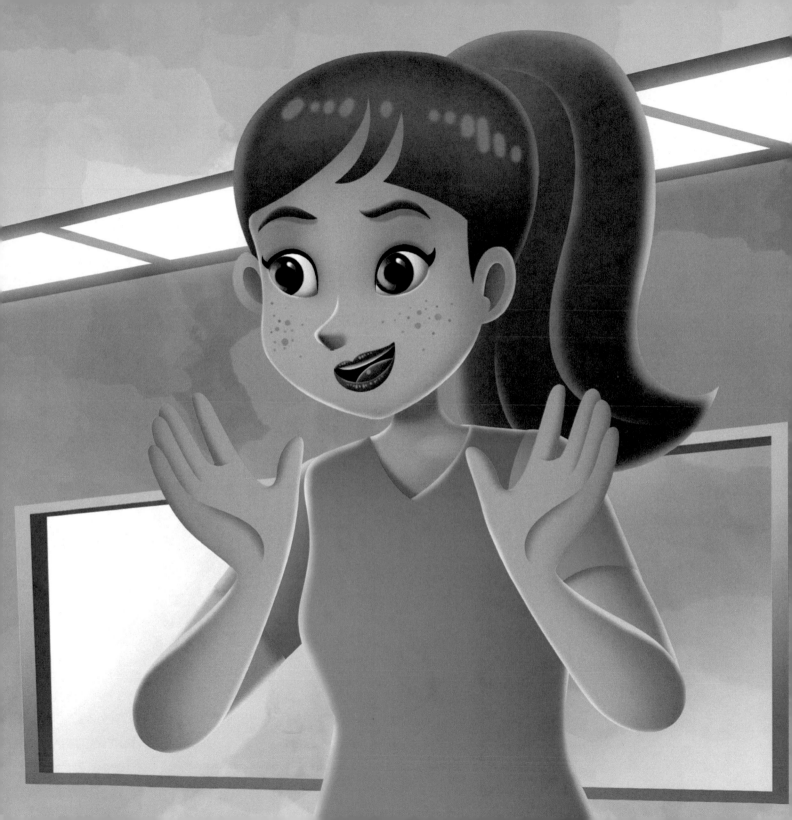

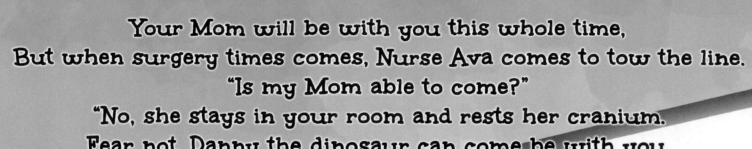

Your Mom will be with you this whole time,
But when surgery times comes, Nurse Ava comes to tow the line.
"Is my Mom able to come?"
"No, she stays in your room and rests her cranium.
Fear not, Danny the dinosaur can come be with you.
Little Man, have I answered all your questions, true?"

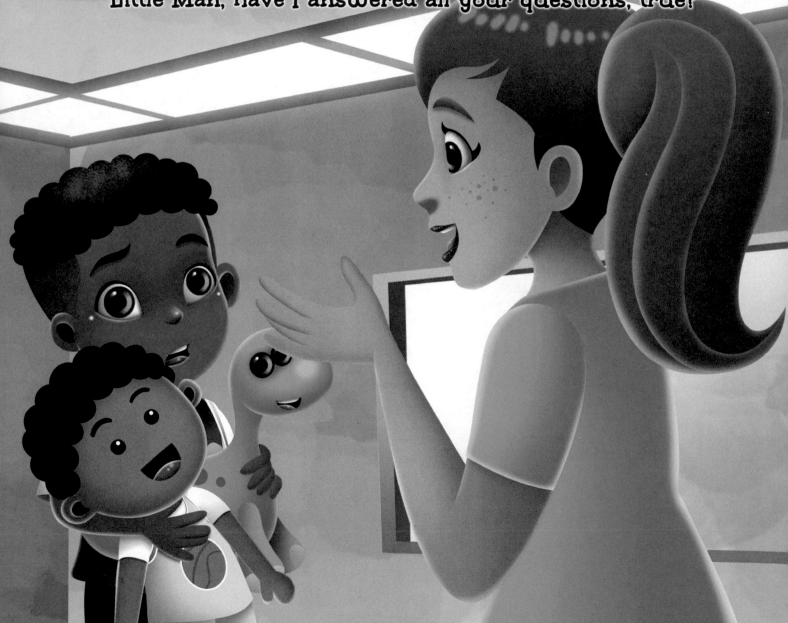

"Mrs. Jen, I am scared."
"That is okay, Little Man, it's normal and you are not spared.
This is because you do not know what to expect,
But you are safe and in good hands, do not object."

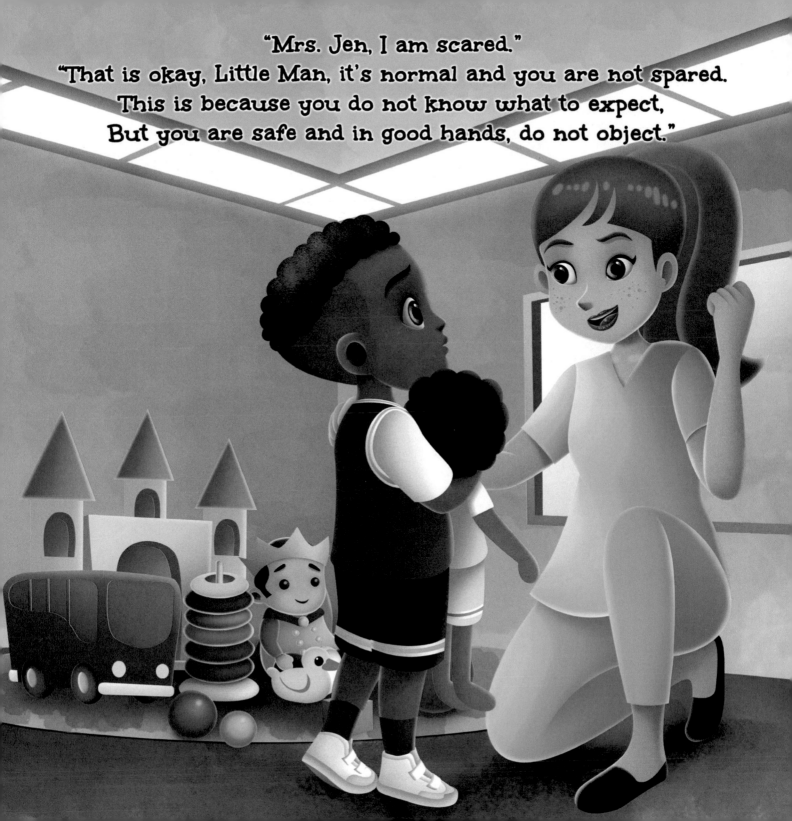

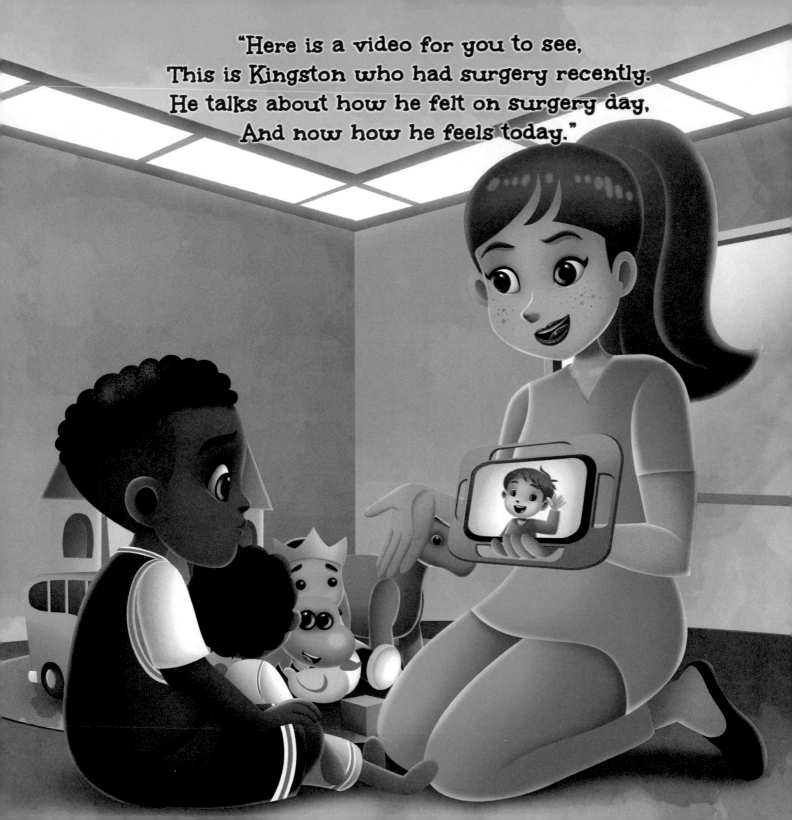

"Here is a video for you to see,
This is Kingston who had surgery recently.
He talks about how he felt on surgery day,
And now how he feels today."

Kingston was smiling and happy.
He talked about surgery day and was not sappy.
He only remembers bright lights and waking up.
Today, Kingston is healthy, and happy and healed up.

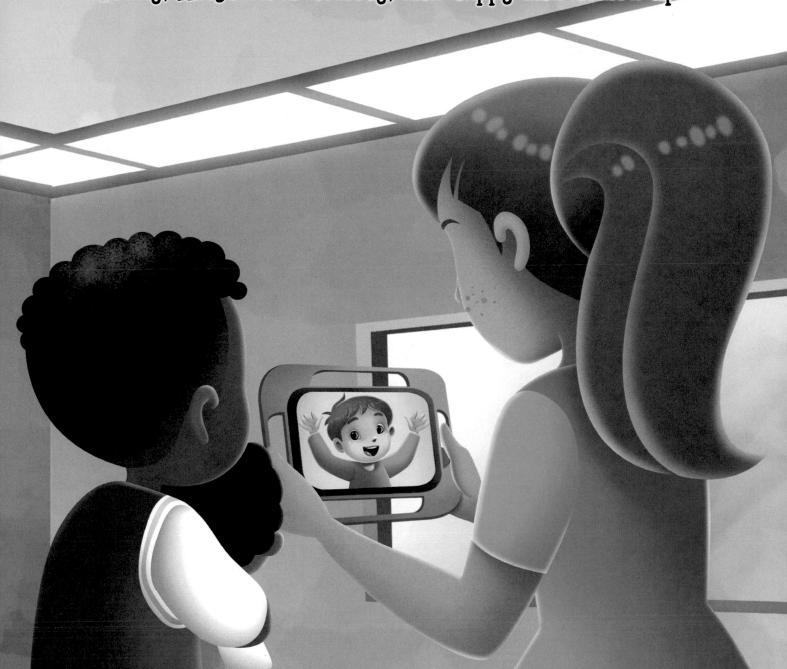

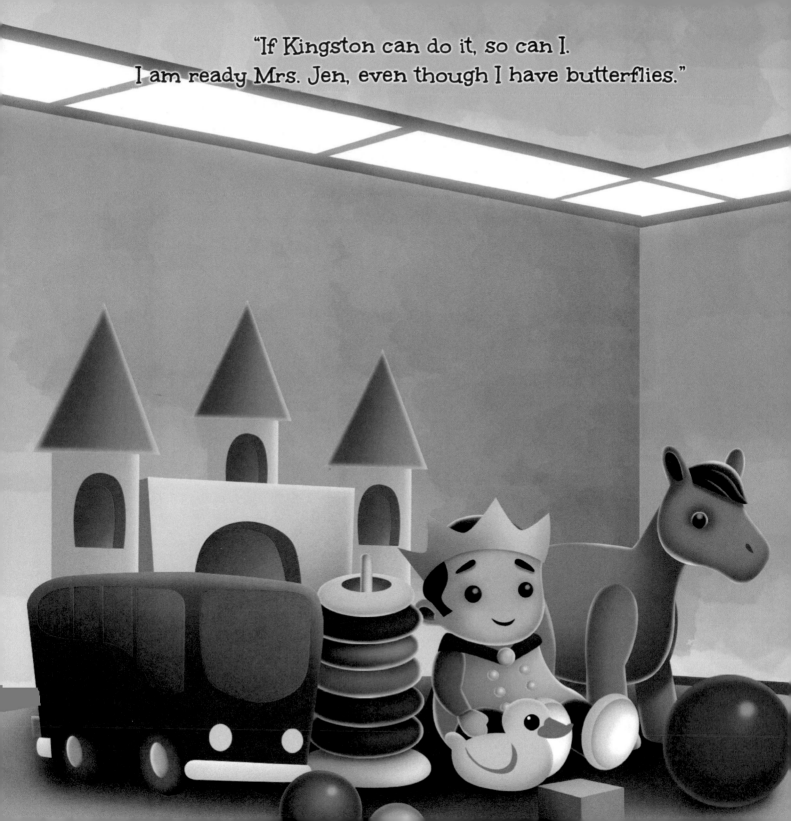

"If Kingston can do it, so can I.
I am ready Mrs. Jen, even though I have butterflies."

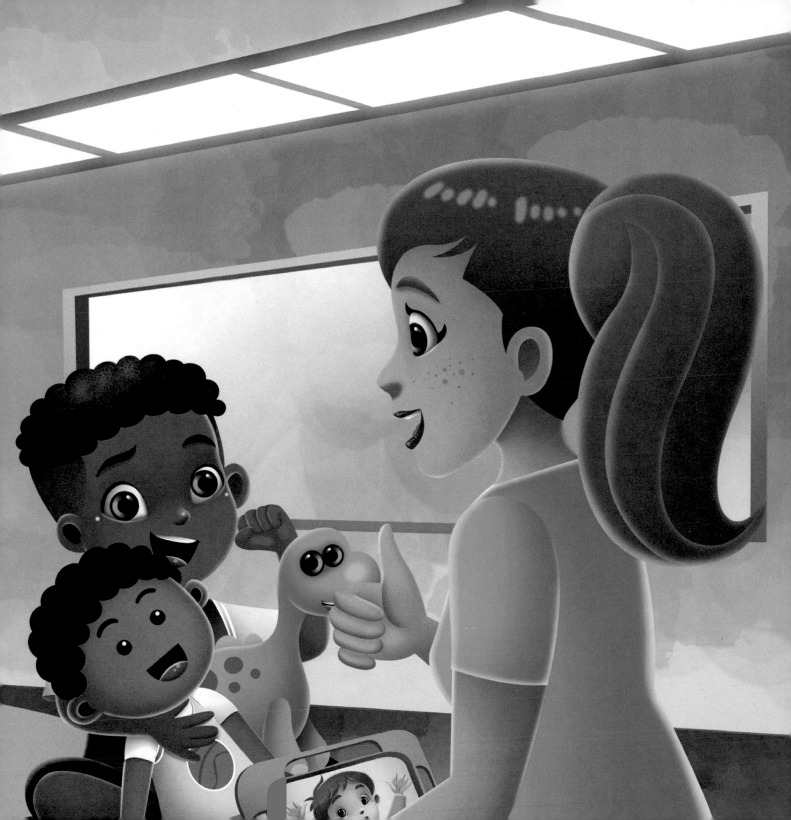

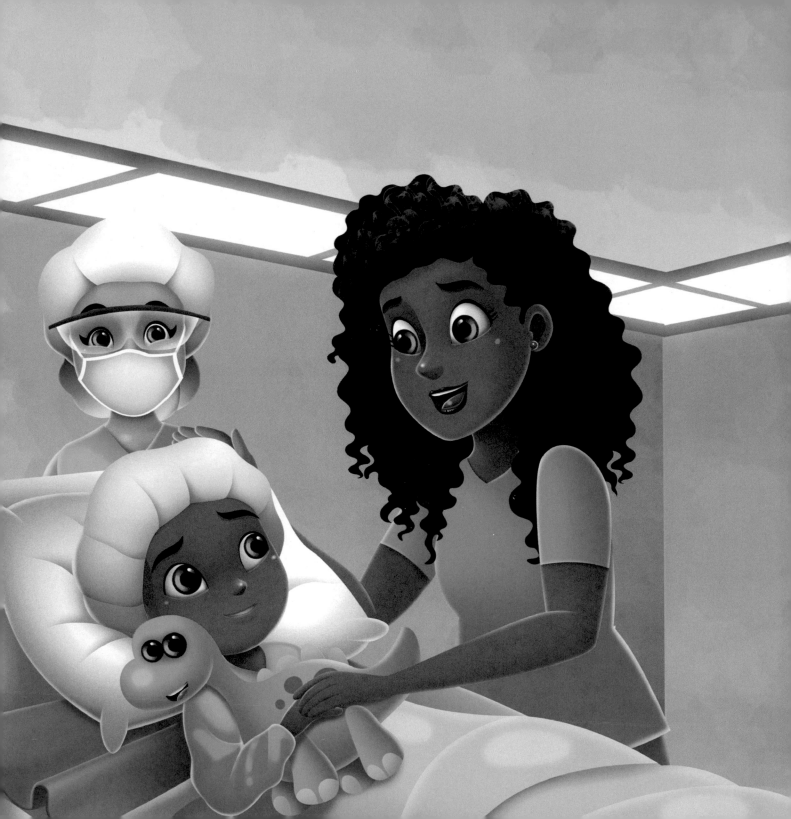

Everything goes just as Ms. Jen described:
Nurse Becky and Dr. Serrano talking all things surgery
Dr. Johanna my anesthesiologist who keeps me sleeping and breathing
Nurse Ava my surgery nurse and
Mr. Tyler my anesthetist for surgery medicine and watching me sleep.
All from the comfort of my bedside.

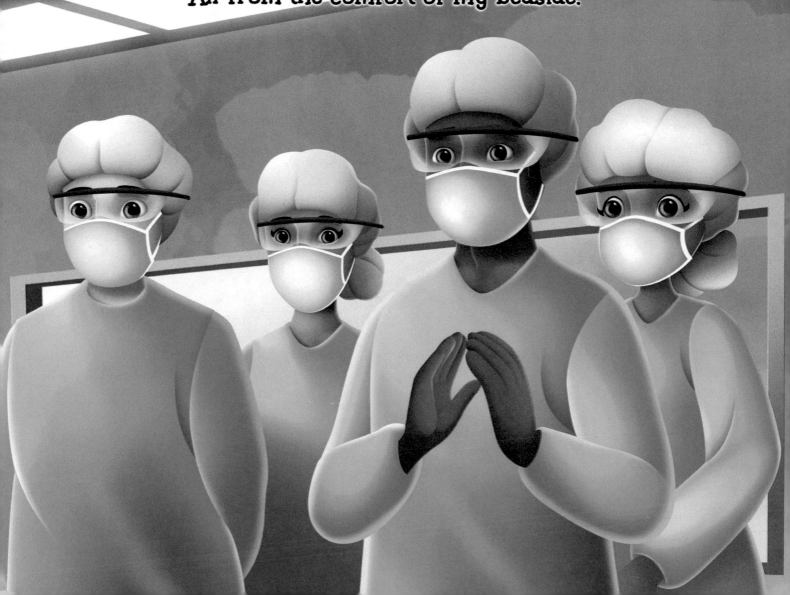

Everyone stops talking and it is time for me to go.
Take those breaks off and get this bed to roll.
Mom gives me a BIG hug and kiss.
"See you soon, Little Man."

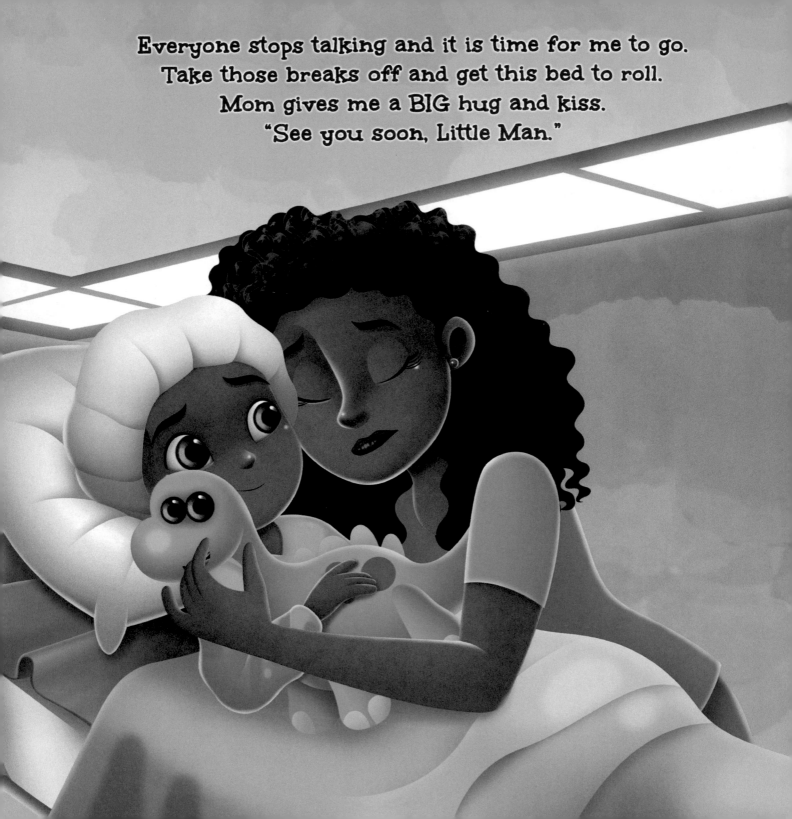

I hold Danny so tight,
And wave my hand for the ride.
We cross a big red line
And cold is the feeling this time.

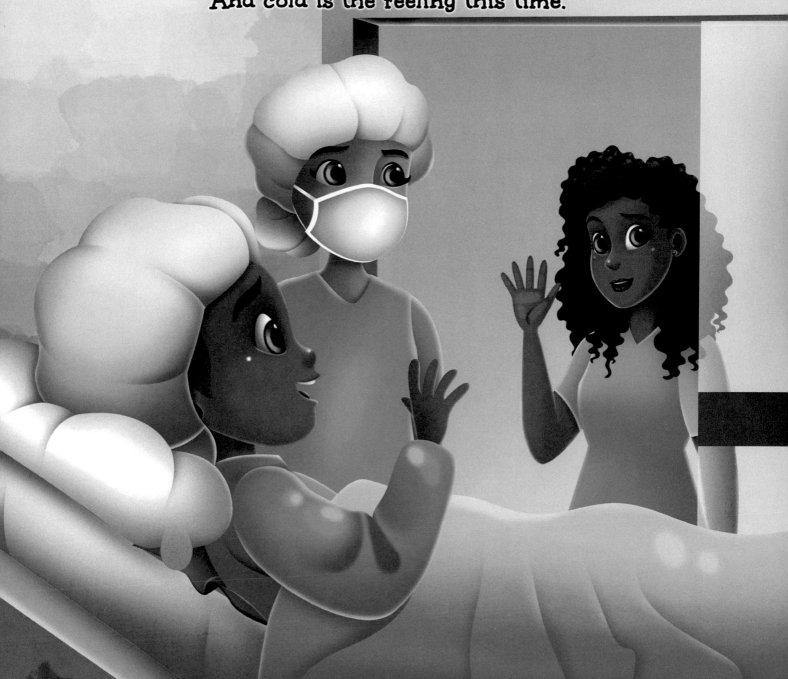

People are in masks with smiling eyes.
They are wearing scrubs and hats like mine—TWINS!

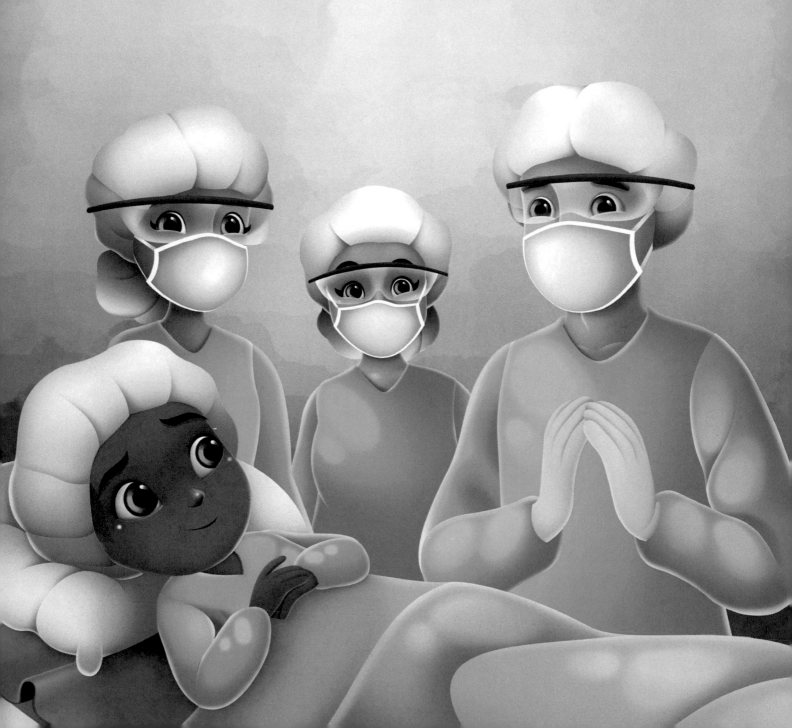

We get to the operating room and Mr. Ed says, "HELLO!
What is your favorite TV show?"
All I say is, "I do not know."
"That is okay, we can go with the flow."

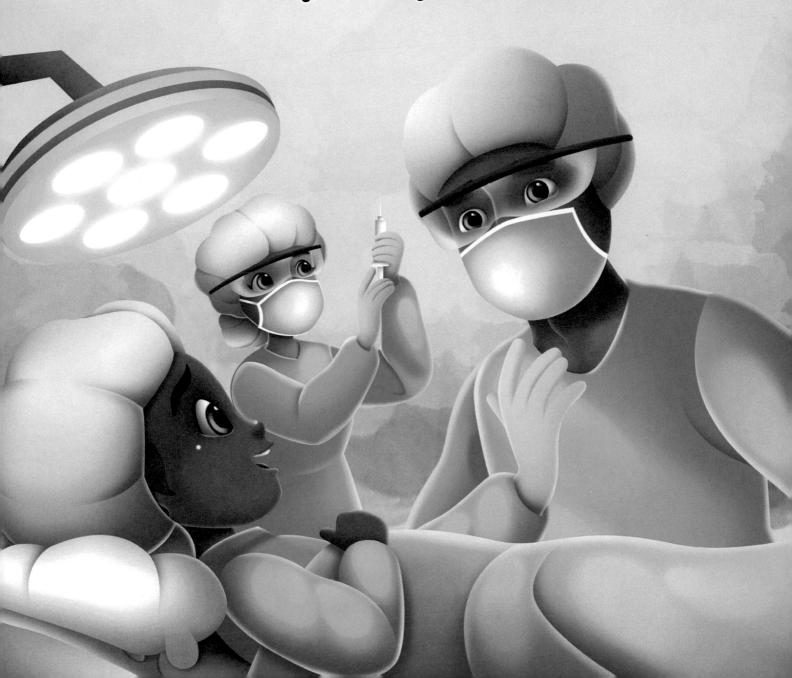

Nurse Ava bundles me up and gets me to the table
"What is your favorite song, Little Man?"
"Beautiful Boy, I am a big fan."

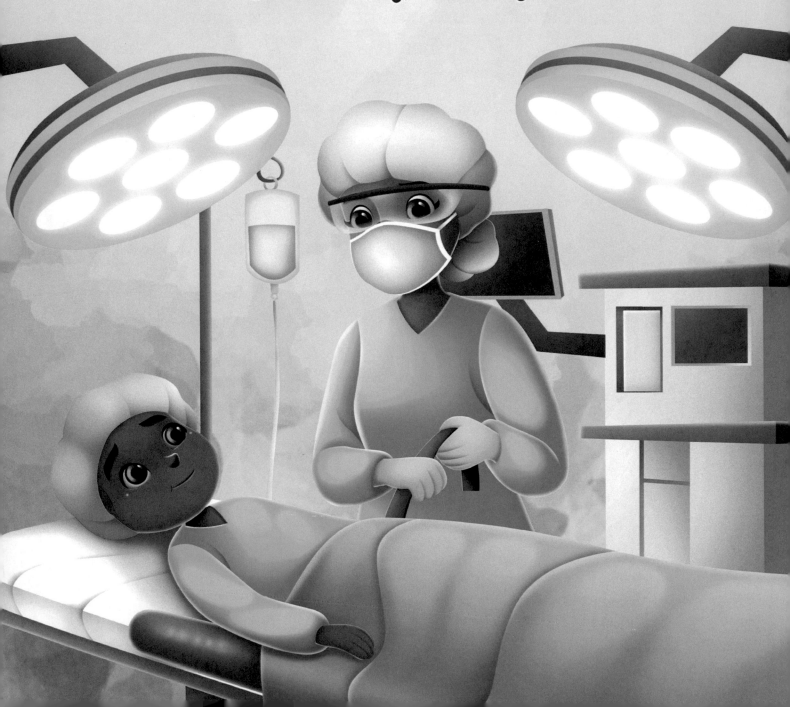

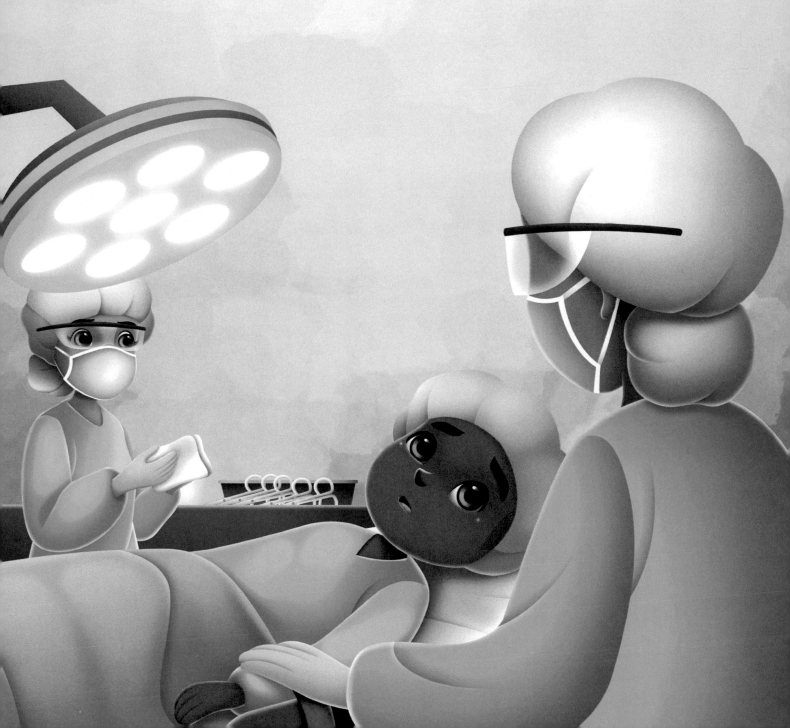

"Nurse Ava, why is it so bright in here?"
"All the better to see you, Little Man."

"Nurse Ava, why is it so cold in here?"
"To keep the germs from coming near."

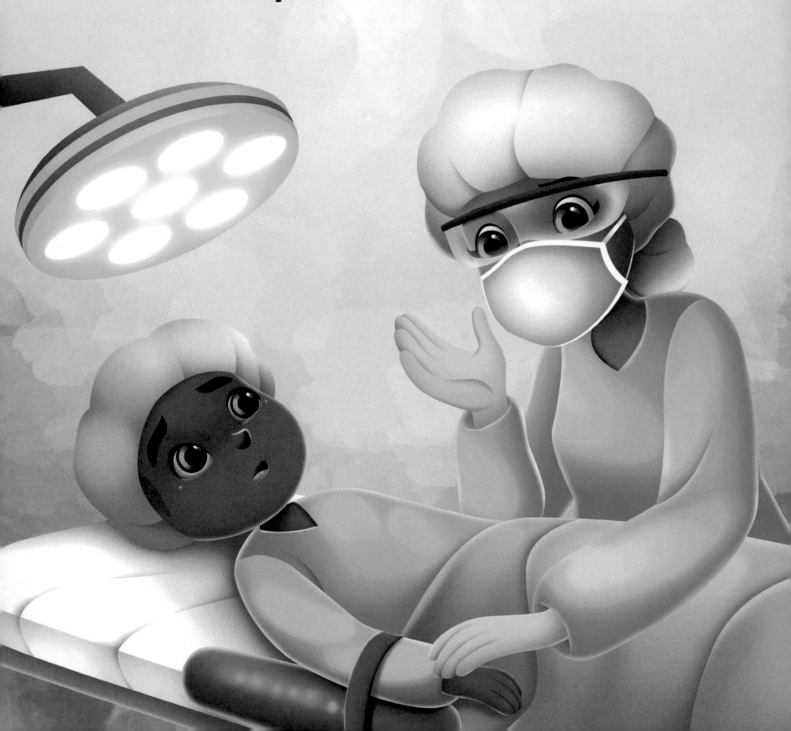

"Nurse Ava I am so tired and my eyes are heavy."
I know Little Man, it is time to be ready."

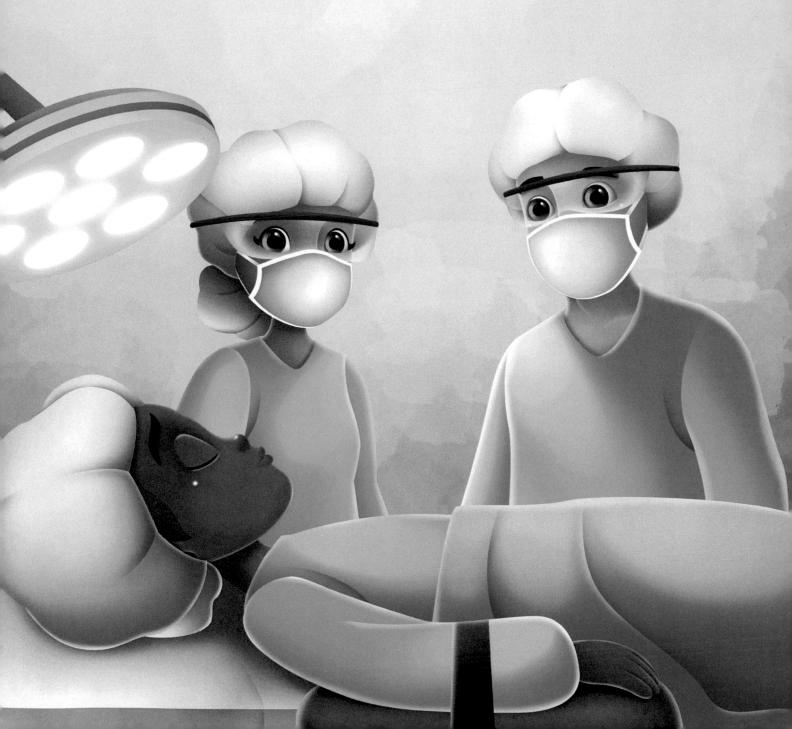

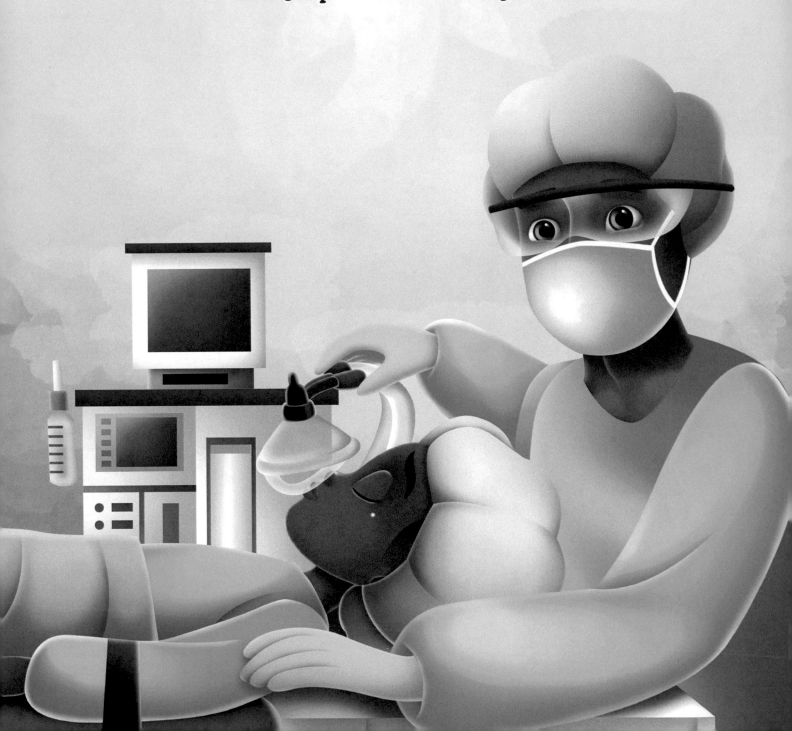

"On your face comes a mask,
Blowing up the balloon is your task."

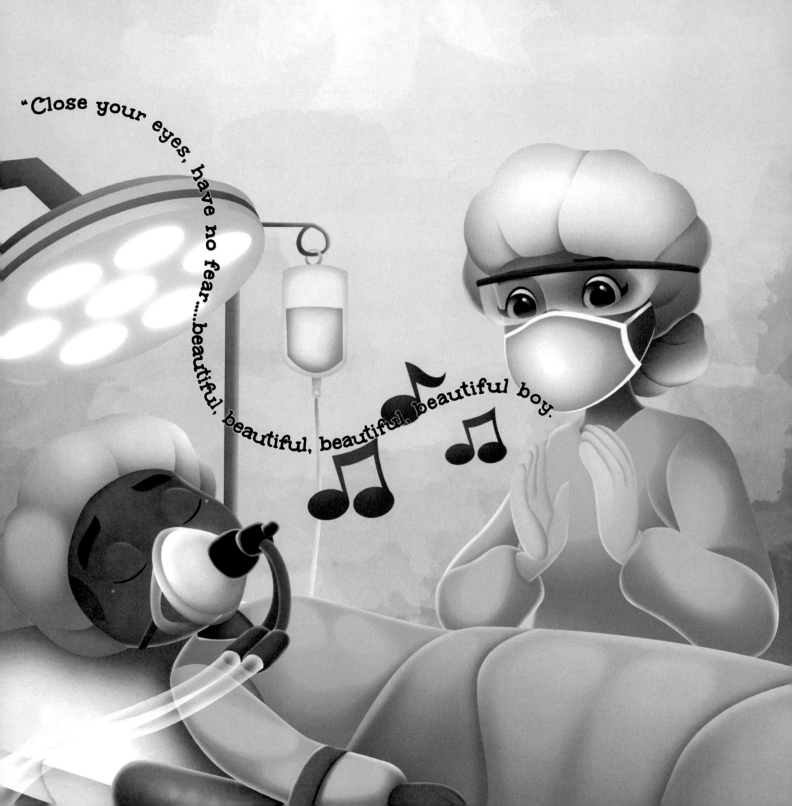

I open my eyes and Mom is by my side.
"Surgery is over, Little Man,
Now give me a BIG kiss."

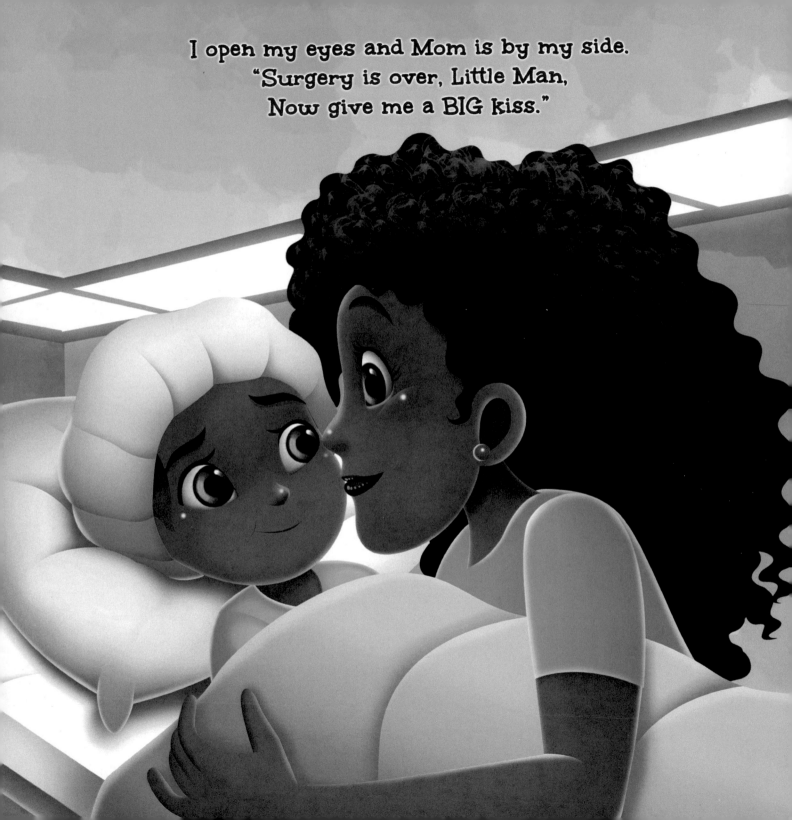

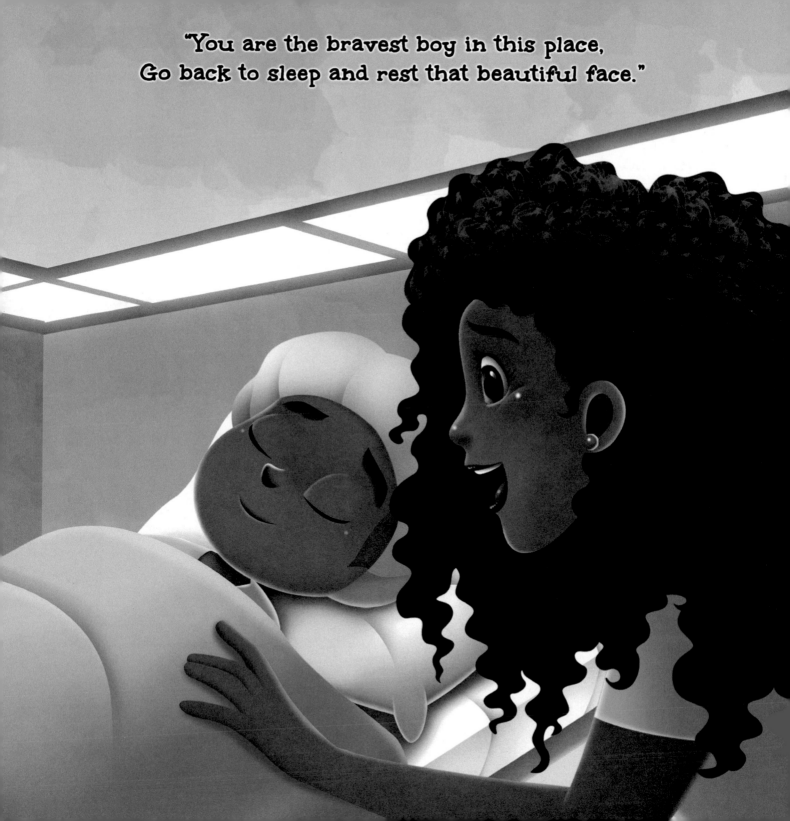

"You are the bravest boy in this place,
Go back to sleep and rest that beautiful face."

Hello Beautiful!

Not sure if you are reading this book because you love the Little Man series or because you will be having surgery. I am an operating room nurse like Nurse Ava. Every day I get to help people and keep them safe on their surgery day. Although it may be scary to have surgery, you have nothing to fear. Facing our fears is the hardest task we will ever do, but being brave and courageous will help you through.

On the day of surgery, you will have many rules to follow like not eating anything before surgery and having to put on a special gown. This is for your safety. You will meet the team that will be with you in the operating room during your surgery and you will be ready for surgery. After that will feel like no time has passed and you will wake up. Don't be afraid to speak up and let your nurse know your needs. And above everything else know everything will be fine.

Hope you have enjoyed this book as much as I have enjoyed writing it.

That's Love,
Erica

If you enjoyed reading this Little Man Story, you might also enjoy reading these other books in the Little Man series and by the author:

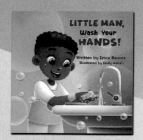 "Little Man Wash Your Hands," is a fun rhyming book that encourages kids to wash their hands.

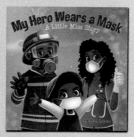 "My Hero Wears a Mask: A Little Miss Story," is a sweet story about a little girl who looks up to her hero, who wears a mask.

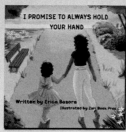 "I Promise to Always Hold Your Hand," is an adorable book about a Mommy and baby girl's promise to each other.

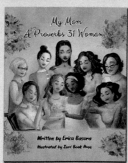 "My Mom a Proverbs 31 Woman," is a beautifully illustrated book that honors mothers everywhere who are hardworking and loving.

Each of these books are sure to please any young reader.

Made in the USA
Las Vegas, NV
25 July 2023

75205695R00024